SPLENECTOMY

A Patient's Guide to Surgery and Recovery

Dr. Bhratri Bhushan,
MD, DM

Copyright © 2025 Dr. Bhratri Bhushan

Copyright © 2025 by Dr. Bhratri Bhushan

All rights reserved. No part of this publication may be reproduced, distributed, or transmitted in any form or by any means, including photocopying, recording, or other electronic or mechanical methods, without the prior written permission of the publisher, except in the case of brief quotations embodied in critical reviews and certain other noncommercial uses permitted by copyright law.

For permission requests, write to the publisher, addressed "Attention: Permissions Coordinator," at the address:

A30, Ananta institute of medical sciences,
Rajsamand, Rajasthan, India 313202
Email: www.bhratri@gmail.com

This work is provided "as is," and the author and the publisher disclaim any and all warranties, express or implied, including any warranties as to accuracy, comprehensiveness, or currency of the content of this work.

To the maximum extent permitted under applicable law, no responsibility is assumed by the publisher for any injury and/or damage to persons or property as a matter of products liability, negligence law or otherwise, or from any reference to or use by any person of this work.

CONTENTS

Title Page
Copyright
Preface
Part 1: Understanding the Spleen   1
What Is the Spleen?   3
When Does the Spleen Become a Problem?   8
Why Might You Need a Splenectomy?   13
Part 2: Preparing for Splenectomy   21
Making the Decision: Is Splenectomy Right for You?   22
What to Expect Before Surgery   29
Vaccinations and Preventive Measures   36
Part 3: The Splenectomy Procedure   43
How Is Splenectomy Performed?   44
Risks and Benefits of Splenectomy   50
Part 4: Life After Splenectomy   57
Your First Days After Surgery   58

Adjusting to Life Without a Spleen	66
Preventing and Managing Infections	72
Follow-Up Care	79
Part 5: Living Well Without a Spleen	87
Diet, Exercise, and Lifestyle Tips	88
Traveling and Special Considerations	93
Children and Splenectomy	98
A letter to the reader	103
About The Author	107

PREFACE

This book is a comprehensive guide to understanding splenectomy—from the reasons it might be necessary to the procedure itself, and ultimately, to life beyond the surgery. Whether you are facing this decision or adjusting to its aftermath, this book offers clear, compassionate insights into every stage of the journey. You will learn about the conditions that lead to splenectomy, the surgical options available, and the steps to recovery, both physical and emotional. Most importantly, this book equips you with the knowledge and strategies to lead a healthy, active life after splenectomy. It is both a resource and a reassurance, designed to empower you with the confidence to take control of your health and embrace your future.

PART 1: UNDERSTANDING THE SPLEEN

WHAT IS THE SPLEEN?

The spleen is a vital organ in the human body, often overlooked until it becomes problematic. Though not as widely known as the heart or lungs, the spleen plays critical roles in immunity, blood filtration, and maintaining overall health. Understanding its location, structure, and functions can provide valuable insights into why the spleen is essential and what happens when it needs to be removed.

Location and Structure

The spleen is a soft, spongy organ located in the upper left side of the abdomen, just beneath the rib cage and close to the stomach. It is roughly fist-sized in adults, weighing about 150-200 grams, though its size can vary depending on health conditions. The spleen is surrounded by a thin capsule of connective tissue that helps protect its delicate inner structures.

Inside, the spleen has two main types of tissue:
1. White Pulp: This area is rich in immune cells, particularly lymphocytes, which play a central role in fighting infections. The white pulp acts as an immune surveillance hub, where pathogens in the blood are identified and attacked.
2. Red Pulp: This tissue is responsible for filtering

and recycling blood. It contains a dense network of blood vessels and specialized cells that remove damaged or old red blood cells and other debris from circulation.

The spleen is highly vascular, receiving blood through the splenic artery and draining it via the splenic vein. Its proximity to the stomach, pancreas, and diaphragm places it in a central position for interacting with various systems.

Functions of the Spleen

The spleen is often compared to a "blood maintenance center" due to its dual role in immunity and blood filtration. Its functions can be categorized into the following:

1. Immune System Support
  - The spleen is a crucial player in the body's immune defense. It acts as a lymphatic organ, where immune cells, particularly white blood cells like lymphocytes and macrophages, are housed and activated.
  - When blood passes through the spleen, it is monitored for the presence of foreign invaders such as bacteria, viruses, and fungi. If pathogens are detected, immune cells in the spleen initiate a rapid response to neutralize them.
  - The white pulp of the spleen acts like a "checkpoint," where antigens (proteins from pathogens) are presented to immune cells,

triggering the production of antibodies and the activation of other defense mechanisms.

- The spleen also stores immune cells and can release them into the bloodstream during infections or inflammatory responses.

2. Blood Filtration and Maintenance

- The spleen acts as a filter for the blood, ensuring that damaged, old, or malformed red blood cells are removed from circulation. Healthy red blood cells continue to deliver oxygen throughout the body, while defective ones are broken down in the spleen.

- Iron and other components from old red blood cells are recycled for use in producing new red blood cells in the bone marrow.

- Platelets, which are involved in blood clotting, are also stored in the spleen. During injuries or emergencies, the spleen can release extra platelets to help control bleeding.

3. Responding to Emergencies

- In times of severe blood loss or infection, the spleen can contract and release stored blood, immune cells, and platelets into circulation, acting as a natural reservoir to help the body recover.

- This ability is particularly important in conditions like trauma or systemic infections, where the body's demand for blood and immune resources increases dramatically.

Role in Immunity

The spleen is one of the body's primary immunological organs. By filtering blood directly rather than lymphatic fluid, it has a unique role in detecting bloodborne infections. Its contributions include:

- Activating the Adaptive Immune System: Lymphocytes in the white pulp are key to mounting specific, long-lasting immune responses. This includes creating memory cells that "remember" pathogens, offering protection against future infections.

- Clearing Bloodborne Pathogens: Specialized cells called macrophages engulf and destroy pathogens in the blood. This ensures that harmful microbes are quickly eliminated before they can spread.

- Producing Antibodies: The spleen aids in generating antibodies that neutralize pathogens and facilitate their removal from the bloodstream.

Role in Blood Filtration

Blood filtration is another cornerstone of the spleen's functions. It operates as a quality-control system, ensuring that only healthy cells circulate:

- Removing Old or Damaged Red Blood Cells: Red blood cells have a lifespan of about 120 days. Once they become old or damaged, they lose flexibility and are trapped in the spleen's fine blood vessels. These cells are then broken down, and their components are recycled.

- Clearing Cellular Debris: The spleen removes debris

from broken cells and any foreign particles that may be circulating in the blood.

- Supporting Bone Marrow Function: By clearing out old cells and debris, the spleen ensures that the bone marrow can focus on producing new, healthy cells without unnecessary strain.

WHEN DOES THE SPLEEN BECOME A PROBLEM?

The spleen is a resilient organ, but like any other part of the body, it can face challenges that impair its ability to function properly. When the spleen becomes damaged, enlarged, or dysfunctional, it can lead to a variety of health problems.

Conditions That Affect the Spleen

The spleen can be affected by a wide range of conditions, from traumatic injuries to systemic diseases. These conditions fall into several categories:

1. Trauma
   - Injuries to the spleen are among the most common causes of acute spleen problems, often resulting from car accidents, sports injuries, or falls.
   - Due to its rich blood supply, a ruptured spleen can lead to life-threatening internal bleeding.
   - Even minor trauma to an already enlarged spleen can cause it to rupture, making conditions like splenomegaly (enlarged spleen) particularly risky.

2. Infections
   - Viral Infections: Certain viral infections, like infectious mononucleosis (caused by the Epstein-Barr virus), can lead to an enlarged spleen.

- Bacterial Infections: Conditions such as endocarditis, tuberculosis, or syphilis can involve the spleen and cause it to become inflamed or dysfunctional.
- Parasitic Infections: Diseases like malaria or leishmaniasis can infect the spleen directly, leading to significant enlargement and compromised function.

3. Cancers and Blood Disorders
- Lymphomas: Hodgkin and non-Hodgkin lymphomas can involve the spleen, as it is a major organ of the lymphatic system.
- Leukemias: Blood cancers like chronic lymphocytic leukemia (CLL) or acute lymphoblastic leukemia (ALL) often affect the spleen due to its role in filtering abnormal blood cells.
- Myeloproliferative Disorders: Conditions such as polycythemia vera or myelofibrosis can cause the spleen to enlarge significantly as it works to compensate for abnormalities in blood production.

4. Splenomegaly (Enlarged Spleen)
- Splenomegaly is a common symptom of various diseases. It occurs when the spleen becomes enlarged, either due to an increase in its workload or infiltration by abnormal cells or substances.
- Causes of splenomegaly include:
  - Chronic liver diseases like cirrhosis, which lead to portal hypertension and congestion of blood in the spleen.
  - Autoimmune diseases such as systemic lupus

erythematosus or rheumatoid arthritis.

- Storage disorders like Gaucher's disease or Niemann-Pick disease, where abnormal substances accumulate in the spleen.

5. Hypersplenism

- Hypersplenism is a condition where an overactive spleen removes too many blood cells (red blood cells, white blood cells, and platelets) from the circulation. This can lead to anemia, leukopenia, and thrombocytopenia.

- It is often associated with splenomegaly and can be caused by underlying infections, cancers, or autoimmune disorders.

6. Ruptured Spleen

- A ruptured spleen is a medical emergency that typically occurs following trauma or in cases of severe splenomegaly.

- The rupture allows blood to leak into the abdominal cavity, causing severe pain, low blood pressure, and shock.

7. Functional Asplenia or Hyposplenism

- In some conditions, the spleen may shrink or lose its ability to function properly, even if it is not physically removed. This is referred to as functional asplenia or hyposplenism.

- Common causes include sickle cell disease (where repeated infarctions damage the spleen) and splenic irradiation for cancer treatment.

Symptoms of Spleen Disorders

Spleen disorders can present with a wide range of symptoms, depending on the underlying cause. Recognizing these symptoms early can help in diagnosing and managing the condition effectively.

1. Pain and Discomfort
   - Abdominal Pain: Pain or discomfort in the upper left side of the abdomen, sometimes radiating to the left shoulder, is a hallmark symptom of spleen problems.
   - Fullness or Bloating: An enlarged spleen can press against the stomach, leading to a sensation of fullness or reduced appetite.

2. Fatigue and Weakness
   - Hypersplenism or an overactive spleen can cause anemia, leading to fatigue, weakness, and shortness of breath.

3. Frequent Infections
   - A dysfunctional spleen may fail to filter bacteria and other pathogens effectively, increasing the risk of recurrent or severe infections.

4. Easy Bruising or Bleeding
   - A reduced platelet count (thrombocytopenia) caused by hypersplenism can lead to easy bruising, nosebleeds, or prolonged bleeding after minor injuries.

5. Jaundice or Pale Skin

- Excessive breakdown of red blood cells by an overactive spleen can lead to jaundice (yellowing of the skin and eyes) or pale skin due to anemia.

6. Unexplained Weight Loss

- Some conditions affecting the spleen, particularly cancers, may cause significant and unexplained weight loss.

7. Swelling or Lump in the Abdomen

- In cases of severe splenomegaly, the spleen may become palpable as a lump in the upper left abdomen.

WHY MIGHT YOU NEED A SPLENECTOMY?

The spleen, a critical organ in your immune and circulatory systems, can sometimes become damaged, diseased, or dysfunctional, necessitating its removal through a procedure called splenectomy. While the spleen plays vital roles in filtering blood and supporting the immune system, its removal is sometimes the best or only option to protect your health. Understanding the conditions that lead to splenectomy and the risks posed by an enlarged or damaged spleen can help patients make informed decisions about their care.

Common Indications for Splenectomy

Several medical conditions can lead to the recommendation for splenectomy. These include trauma, blood disorders, infections, cancers, and congenital abnormalities. Below are the most common scenarios where splenectomy may be necessary:

1. Trauma
   - The spleen is one of the most commonly injured organs in abdominal trauma due to its soft texture and rich blood supply.
   - Blunt trauma from car accidents, sports injuries, or falls can cause the spleen to rupture, leading to

life-threatening internal bleeding.

- In cases where bleeding cannot be controlled or the spleen is severely damaged, immediate splenectomy may be required to save the patient's life.

2. Immune Thrombocytopenic Purpura (ITP)

- ITP is an autoimmune disorder in which the immune system mistakenly attacks platelets, the cells responsible for blood clotting. This leads to low platelet counts and an increased risk of bleeding.

- The spleen plays a role in destroying platelets targeted by the immune system. Removing the spleen can help reduce platelet destruction and increase platelet counts in patients whose ITP does not respond to medications like steroids or immunoglobulins.

- Splenectomy is not the first-line treatment for ITP but may be recommended for chronic cases.

3. Hereditary Spherocytosis

- This genetic condition affects the structure of red blood cells, causing them to be sphere-shaped instead of the normal disc shape. These abnormal cells are more prone to destruction, especially in the spleen.

- The excessive breakdown of red blood cells leads to anemia, jaundice, and an enlarged spleen.

- Splenectomy is often performed to improve red blood cell survival and alleviate symptoms, particularly in moderate to severe cases.

4. Splenic Abscess
- A splenic abscess is a rare but serious condition in which pus collects in the spleen due to an infection. It can occur from bloodborne infections, trauma, or other sources of sepsis.
- Patients with a splenic abscess may experience fever, abdominal pain, and general malaise. If the abscess does not respond to antibiotics or drainage, splenectomy may be necessary to remove the infected tissue.

5. Splenic Cysts or Tumors
- While benign cysts and tumors of the spleen are uncommon, they can sometimes grow large enough to cause discomfort, rupture, or impair the spleen's function.
- In cases where cysts or tumors pose a risk of rupture or become symptomatic, splenectomy may be recommended.

6. Cancers Involving the Spleen
- The spleen can be affected by certain cancers, such as:
    - Lymphomas (Hodgkin and non-Hodgkin): These cancers of the lymphatic system often involve the spleen.
    - Leukemias: Chronic lymphocytic leukemia (CLL) or acute lymphoblastic leukemia (ALL) can infiltrate the spleen, causing it to enlarge and become dysfunctional.
    - Metastatic Cancer: Rarely, cancers from other

parts of the body may spread to the spleen.
- In such cases, splenectomy may be performed to control disease progression, alleviate symptoms, or improve response to other treatments like chemotherapy.

7. Thrombotic or Hematologic Disorders
- Disorders that affect blood clotting or red blood cell survival may involve the spleen:
  - Thalassemia: In severe forms of this inherited blood disorder, the spleen may enlarge as it tries to filter defective red blood cells. Removing the spleen can help alleviate symptoms.
  - Sickle Cell Disease: Chronic damage to the spleen in sickle cell disease may lead to functional asplenia or necessitate splenectomy in specific situations.
  - Myeloproliferative Disorders: Conditions like myelofibrosis can cause massive spleen enlargement and associated discomfort, leading to splenectomy in advanced cases.

8. Enlarged Spleen (Splenomegaly)
- Splenomegaly can occur due to various underlying conditions, including infections, liver diseases, or cancers.
- While splenomegaly itself is not always an indication for splenectomy, it may become necessary if the enlarged spleen:
  - Causes severe pain or discomfort.
  - Compresses nearby organs like the stomach, leading to early satiety or difficulty eating.

- Becomes at risk for rupture, even with minor trauma.

Understanding the Risks of an Enlarged or Damaged Spleen

An enlarged or damaged spleen poses several risks that can significantly impact a person's health. These risks highlight why splenectomy may be necessary in some cases:

1. Rupture and Internal Bleeding
- An enlarged spleen is more fragile and prone to rupture, even with minor trauma. Rupture can lead to massive internal bleeding, which is a medical emergency.
- Patients with splenomegaly must often avoid contact sports or activities that increase the risk of abdominal trauma.

2. Increased Blood Cell Destruction
- An overactive spleen (hypersplenism) may destroy healthy blood cells in addition to abnormal ones. This can result in:
  - Anemia: Low red blood cell count, leading to fatigue, weakness, and shortness of breath.
  - Leukopenia: Low white blood cell count, increasing susceptibility to infections.
  - Thrombocytopenia: Low platelet count, leading to easy bruising and excessive bleeding.

3. Compression of Nearby Organs
- An enlarged spleen can press on neighboring

organs, causing:

- Stomach Compression: Leading to a feeling of fullness after eating small amounts.
- Diaphragm Compression: Causing difficulty breathing in severe cases.

4. Impaired Immune Function

- A damaged spleen may fail to perform its immunological role effectively, leaving the body more vulnerable to infections, particularly those caused by encapsulated bacteria like Streptococcus pneumoniae, Haemophilus influenzae, and Neisseria meningitidis.

Weighing the Benefits and Risks of Splenectomy

Splenectomy is a major surgery that is typically reserved for cases where the benefits outweigh the risks. The decision to remove the spleen depends on:
- The severity of the underlying condition.
- The impact of the spleen disorder on the patient's quality of life.
- The risk of complications from leaving the spleen untreated.

While the body can adapt to life without a spleen, patients who undergo splenectomy must take lifelong precautions to reduce the risk of infections. These include:
- Regular vaccinations (e.g., pneumococcal, meningococcal, and Haemophilus influenzae type B

vaccines).
- Preventive antibiotics for high-risk situations.
- Prompt treatment of any suspected infections.

PART 2: PREPARING FOR SPLENECTOMY

MAKING THE DECISION: IS SPLENECTOMY RIGHT FOR YOU?

Deciding whether to undergo splenectomy, the surgical removal of the spleen, is a complex process that involves careful consideration of the benefits, risks, and alternatives. While splenectomy can resolve certain medical conditions, it also comes with lifelong implications for the immune system. Doctors weigh many factors when recommending this procedure, and understanding the decision-making process can help you feel confident and informed about your treatment.

How Doctors Decide on Splenectomy

Splenectomy is not usually the first-line treatment for most conditions. Doctors carefully evaluate the necessity of the procedure based on the patient's condition, the potential benefits, and the risks involved. Here are the key factors that guide their decision:

1. Underlying Medical Condition
The primary reason for recommending splenectomy is the presence of a condition that either directly affects the spleen or requires its removal to improve overall health. Common conditions include:
   - Trauma: A ruptured spleen from an accident

is often an emergency that necessitates immediate removal to prevent life-threatening internal bleeding.

- Blood Disorders: Chronic conditions like immune thrombocytopenic purpura (ITP), hereditary spherocytosis, or thalassemia may warrant splenectomy if other treatments fail.

- Infections or Abscesses: Severe infections or abscesses in the spleen that do not respond to antibiotics or drainage may require removal to prevent further complications.

- Cancers: Lymphomas, leukemias, or metastases involving the spleen may lead to splenectomy as part of the treatment plan.

- Enlarged Spleen (Splenomegaly): If splenomegaly is causing pain, compression of nearby organs, or excessive blood cell destruction (hypersplenism), splenectomy may be necessary.

2. Severity of Symptoms

Doctors assess the severity of your symptoms to determine whether splenectomy is the most appropriate intervention. Indications include:

- Persistent pain or discomfort from an enlarged spleen.
- Severe anemia, thrombocytopenia, or leukopenia due to hypersplenism that significantly impacts quality of life.
- Recurrent or uncontrolled infections due to splenic dysfunction.

3. Response to Non-Surgical Treatments

Splenectomy is generally considered only after less invasive treatments have been tried and found to be ineffective or unsuitable. For example:

- In ITP, corticosteroids, immunoglobulins, or newer medications like thrombopoietin receptor agonists are typically the first line of treatment. Splenectomy is reserved for patients with chronic, refractory ITP.

- In hereditary spherocytosis, splenectomy is often delayed until symptoms become moderate to severe, especially in children, to minimize risks.

4. Risk of Complications

Doctors carefully evaluate the risks of splenectomy versus the risks of leaving the spleen untreated. A damaged or overactive spleen can lead to serious complications, such as:

- Life-threatening bleeding from a ruptured spleen.
- Severe infections due to splenic abscesses or impaired immune function.
- Worsening anemia, thrombocytopenia, or other blood disorders caused by hypersplenism.

In these cases, the benefits of removing the spleen often outweigh the risks associated with the procedure.

5. Patient's Overall Health

A patient's general health and ability to tolerate surgery are critical factors in the decision. Conditions like advanced age, heart disease, or other chronic illnesses may increase surgical risks. Doctors also consider:

- Immune Status: The spleen plays a central role in the immune system, so patients must be vaccinated against certain infections before surgery.

- Liver Function: In patients with cirrhosis and portal hypertension, splenectomy can increase the risk of complications like thrombosis, requiring a more cautious approach.

6. Emergency Versus Elective Surgery
The urgency of the situation influences the decision-making process. Splenectomy performed in an emergency (e.g., for a ruptured spleen) often leaves less time for preoperative planning. In contrast, elective splenectomy allows for thorough preparation, including vaccinations and optimization of health conditions.

Alternative Treatments and
When They Might Work

Splenectomy is not the only option for managing spleen-related conditions. Depending on the diagnosis, several non-surgical or less invasive treatments may be effective. Exploring these alternatives can help patients avoid the long-term consequences of splenectomy, such as increased susceptibility to infections.

1. Medications
   - Immune Suppressants and Steroids:

- Conditions like ITP often respond well to corticosteroids (e.g., prednisone), which reduce the immune system's attack on platelets.
- Immunosuppressants or biologic agents like rituximab can also modulate the immune response in refractory cases.
- Erythropoiesis-Stimulating Agents:
- In conditions like anemia due to hereditary spherocytosis, medications that stimulate red blood cell production can help alleviate symptoms.
- Thrombopoietin Receptor Agonists:
- Drugs like eltrombopag or romiplostim can increase platelet production in ITP patients, reducing the need for splenectomy.

2. Vaccinations and Prophylactic Antibiotics

- In patients with functional asplenia or splenic dysfunction, regular vaccinations and prophylactic antibiotics can prevent severe infections. This is often sufficient to manage mild cases without resorting to surgery.

3. Splenic Embolization

- In some cases, partial splenic embolization (blocking blood flow to a portion of the spleen) can reduce the organ's size and function without completely removing it.
- This procedure may be an option for patients with hypersplenism or splenic trauma who are not candidates for surgery.

4. Drainage of Abscesses

- For splenic abscesses, image-guided drainage may be attempted before considering splenectomy. Antibiotics are used alongside drainage to treat the infection.

5. Monitoring and Lifestyle Adjustments
- For mild splenomegaly or conditions with minimal symptoms, doctors may recommend watchful waiting, along with lifestyle changes to reduce risks. These might include:
   - Avoiding contact sports or activities that increase the risk of abdominal trauma.
   - Regular monitoring of blood counts and spleen size.

6. Gene Therapy and Emerging Treatments
- For inherited conditions like thalassemia or hereditary spherocytosis, emerging treatments like gene therapy or bone marrow transplantation may offer alternatives to splenectomy in the future.

Factors Influencing the Choice of Alternatives

While alternatives to splenectomy can be effective, they are not suitable for everyone. The decision depends on:
- Severity of the Condition: Advanced or refractory conditions may leave no choice but splenectomy.
- Patient's Age: Children are more likely to be managed with non-surgical treatments or delayed

splenectomy to minimize long-term risks.

- Effectiveness of Non-Surgical Options: If medications or procedures fail to control symptoms or prevent complications, surgery becomes the next step.

Balancing the Benefits and Risks

Ultimately, the decision to undergo splenectomy involves weighing the benefits of resolving the underlying condition against the risks of surgery and life without a spleen. Key considerations include:

- The likelihood of improving quality of life and preventing complications.
- The patient's ability to adapt to life without a spleen, including following preventive measures like vaccinations and infection monitoring.
- The availability and effectiveness of alternative treatments.

By working closely with their healthcare team, patients can make informed decisions about whether splenectomy is the right choice for their unique circumstances.

WHAT TO EXPECT BEFORE SURGERY

Undergoing splenectomy, the surgical removal of the spleen, is a significant medical procedure that requires careful preparation. Both pre-operative evaluations and physical and mental readiness play critical roles in ensuring the best possible outcomes. Knowing what to expect before surgery can alleviate anxiety and help you feel more confident about the process.

Pre-Operative Tests and Evaluations

Before proceeding with a splenectomy, your medical team will conduct a series of tests and evaluations to ensure you are healthy enough for surgery and to optimize your care. These tests are designed to assess your overall health, identify any risks, and plan for any necessary interventions before or during the procedure.

1. Medical History and Physical Examination
   - Your doctor will review your complete medical history, including:
     - Any underlying medical conditions (e.g., diabetes, hypertension, or clotting disorders).
     - Previous surgeries and reactions to anesthesia.
     - Current medications, including over-the-counter drugs, supplements, and herbal remedies.
     - Allergies, especially to medications or latex.

- A thorough physical examination will focus on your abdomen, where the spleen is located, and any symptoms like pain, fullness, or tenderness.

2. Blood Tests

- Complete Blood Count (CBC): This test evaluates your red and white blood cells and platelets. It can reveal anemia, thrombocytopenia, or infections.
- Coagulation Profile: Tests like PT, INR, and aPTT assess your blood's ability to clot, which is vital to minimize bleeding risks during and after surgery.
- Liver and Kidney Function Tests: These help ensure your organs are functioning well enough to handle surgery and anesthesia.
- Blood Typing and Crossmatching: In case you need a blood transfusion during surgery, your blood type will be determined, and compatible blood will be prepared.

3. Imaging Studies

- Ultrasound or CT Scan: These imaging tests provide detailed pictures of your spleen and surrounding organs. They help confirm the size of the spleen, identify abnormalities, and assess the proximity to other structures.
- MRI (if needed): Occasionally, an MRI may be ordered for more precise imaging, especially if there are concerns about nearby blood vessels or tumors.

4. Vaccination Assessment

- The spleen plays a critical role in fighting infections, particularly those caused by encapsulated bacteria like Streptococcus pneumoniae, Haemophilus influenzae, and Neisseria meningitidis.

- Before surgery, your doctor will ensure you are vaccinated against these pathogens to protect you from post-splenectomy infections. Vaccines typically administered include:
    - Pneumococcal Vaccine (PCV13 and PPSV23)
    - Meningococcal Vaccine (MenACWY and MenB)
    - Haemophilus Influenzae Type B (Hib) Vaccine
- These vaccines are ideally given at least 2–4 weeks before an elective splenectomy. For emergency surgeries, vaccines are administered shortly after recovery.

5. Pre-Anesthesia Evaluation
- An anesthesiologist will evaluate you to determine the safest approach to anesthesia during surgery. This evaluation includes:
    - A review of your medical history and prior reactions to anesthesia.
    - Physical examination of your airway, heart, and lungs.
    - Recommendations regarding fasting and medications on the day of surgery.

6. Cardiac and Respiratory Tests
- For patients with heart or lung conditions, additional tests like an ECG (electrocardiogram) or pulmonary function tests may be required.
- These tests help assess your ability to tolerate surgery and anesthesia.

7. Specialist Consultations
- Depending on your condition, your doctor may involve specialists such as hematologists (for blood disorders), oncologists (for cancers), or infectious disease experts (for infections or vaccination planning).

Preparing Mentally and Physically for the Procedure

Mental and physical preparation is just as important as medical evaluations. Taking the right steps before surgery can improve your recovery and help you feel more in control of the process.

1. Physical Preparation

a. Diet and Nutrition
- Healthy Eating: Focus on a balanced diet rich in vitamins, minerals, and proteins to support healing and boost your immune system.
- Iron Supplements: If you have anemia, your doctor may recommend iron or folic acid supplements to optimize your red blood cell levels before surgery.
- Fasting: You will be instructed to stop eating and drinking for a specific period (usually 8–12 hours) before surgery to reduce the risk of complications under anesthesia.

b. Medication Adjustments
- Blood Thinners: If you are on blood-thinning

medications like aspirin, warfarin, or clopidogrel, you may need to stop these several days before surgery to reduce the risk of bleeding.

- Other Medications: Your doctor may adjust medications for diabetes, high blood pressure, or other chronic conditions. Always follow their instructions carefully.

- Prophylactic Antibiotics: You may be given antibiotics to reduce the risk of infections during surgery.

c. Smoking and Alcohol

- Quit Smoking: Smoking can impair healing and increase the risk of lung complications after surgery. If possible, quit smoking at least a few weeks before the procedure.

- Limit Alcohol: Reduce alcohol consumption to support liver function and overall health.

d. Exercise and Fitness

- Staying active before surgery can improve your stamina and speed up your recovery. Light to moderate exercise, as approved by your doctor, is encouraged.

2. Mental and Emotional Preparation

a. Educate Yourself

- Learn about the procedure, including how it is performed, what to expect during recovery, and the potential risks and benefits. Understanding the process can reduce fear of the unknown.

- Ask your doctor any questions you have about

the surgery or post-operative care.

b. Manage Anxiety

- Feeling nervous before surgery is normal. Consider relaxation techniques like deep breathing, meditation, or guided imagery to calm your mind.

- Talking to a therapist or counselor can also help if you are feeling overwhelmed.

c. Support System

- Arrange for a trusted family member or friend to accompany you to the hospital and assist you during your recovery period.

- Share your concerns with loved ones and let them support you emotionally.

d. Advance Planning

- Prepare for your hospital stay by packing comfortable clothes, personal hygiene items, and any necessary documents.

- If you are a caregiver or have dependents, arrange for someone to help with household tasks and responsibilities while you recover.

3. Pre-Surgery Checklist

- Confirm Surgery Time: Your hospital or surgical center will provide you with the exact time to arrive.

- Fasting Instructions: Follow guidelines about when to stop eating and drinking.

- Clothing: Wear loose, comfortable clothing to the hospital.

- Personal Items: Leave valuables at home, but bring essentials like ID, insurance information, and a list of medications.

- Transportation: Arrange for someone to drive you home after the procedure.

VACCINATIONS AND PREVENTIVE MEASURES

In the context of a splenectomy, the importance of vaccinations and preventive measures cannot be overstated. The spleen is a vital part of the immune system, playing a key role in protecting the body against certain types of infections, particularly those caused by encapsulated bacteria. Without a functioning spleen, the body becomes more vulnerable to serious and life-threatening infections. While some aspects of this topic were introduced earlier, it requires further exploration to ensure clarity and a deeper understanding of why these measures are critical before and after surgery.

Importance of Pre-Splenectomy Vaccinations

Pre-splenectomy vaccinations are an essential component of preparing for surgery. They help bolster the immune system against specific pathogens that the spleen typically helps defend against. Since the removal of the spleen compromises the body's ability to combat these infections, vaccines provide an added layer of protection.

Key Vaccines Administered Before Splenectomy

1. Pneumococcal Vaccine
- The pneumococcus bacteria (Streptococcus pneumoniae) is one of the most significant threats to individuals without a spleen. It can cause severe infections such as pneumonia, meningitis, and bloodstream infections (sepsis).
- Two types of pneumococcal vaccines are typically recommended:
   - PCV13 (Prevnar 13): Protects against 13 strains of pneumococcus.
   - PPSV23 (Pneumovax 23): Provides broader protection against 23 strains of the bacteria.
- The PCV13 vaccine is usually administered first, followed by PPSV23 after an interval of at least 8 weeks. This sequential approach ensures maximum immune response.

2. Meningococcal Vaccine
- Neisseria meningitidis, the bacterium responsible for meningococcal disease, can cause meningitis and septicemia, both of which are life-threatening.
- Two types of meningococcal vaccines are recommended:
   - MenACWY (Menactra or Menveo): Protects against meningococcal serogroups A, C, W, and Y.
   - MenB (Bexsero or Trumenba): Protects against serogroup B, which is not covered by MenACWY.
- Both vaccines should be given prior to splenectomy if time allows, with MenB requiring a two-dose schedule.

3. Haemophilus Influenzae Type B (Hib) Vaccine

- Haemophilus influenzae type B was once a leading cause of serious infections like meningitis and epiglottitis, especially in children. Although the incidence of Hib infections has decreased significantly due to widespread childhood vaccination, individuals without a spleen remain at higher risk.
- A single dose of the Hib vaccine is recommended for adults who have not previously received it.

Timing of Vaccinations

- Ideally, vaccinations should be administered at least 2–4 weeks before an elective splenectomy. This allows the body to develop a robust immune response before the surgery.
- In emergency splenectomies, where prior vaccination is not possible, the vaccines are given as soon as possible post-surgery, usually within the first two weeks of recovery.

Preventing Infections Post-Surgery

After a splenectomy, the immune system is permanently altered, and lifelong vigilance is required to prevent infections. This includes additional vaccinations, prophylactic antibiotics, and lifestyle modifications.

1. Additional Vaccinations

While pre-splenectomy vaccinations cover major risks, certain additional vaccines and booster doses

are needed over time to maintain protection:
- Annual Influenza Vaccine:
  - The flu can weaken the immune system and make patients more susceptible to secondary bacterial infections like pneumonia.
- COVID-19 Vaccine:
  - Asplenic patients are at higher risk of severe illness from COVID-19, so full vaccination and booster doses are recommended.
- Hepatitis Vaccines:
  - Hepatitis A and B vaccines may be advised, especially if you are at risk due to travel or lifestyle factors.
- Booster Doses:
  - Pneumococcal and meningococcal vaccines require periodic boosters:
    - PPSV23 booster every 5 years.
    - MenACWY booster every 5 years.
- Other Travel-Related Vaccines:
  - If traveling to regions with malaria or other endemic diseases, additional vaccines or prophylaxis may be needed.

2. Prophylactic Antibiotics

To further reduce the risk of serious infections, many doctors prescribe prophylactic antibiotics, particularly in the first two years following splenectomy, or for younger patients under the age of 16. Common recommendations include:
- Penicillin V or Amoxicillin: Low-dose antibiotics taken daily to prevent bacterial infections.

- For patients allergic to penicillin, alternatives like erythromycin or azithromycin may be prescribed.
- Prophylaxis may be lifelong for some high-risk individuals, such as those with a history of severe infections.

3. Emergency Antibiotics

Asplenic patients should keep a supply of emergency antibiotics at home or with them while traveling. If signs of infection, such as fever, chills, or severe malaise, occur, they should start antibiotics immediately and seek medical attention.

4. Recognizing and Responding to Infections

Without a spleen, the body's response to infections may be delayed or muted. It's crucial for patients to:

- Be vigilant for symptoms like fever, chills, shortness of breath, or confusion, as these may indicate serious infections like sepsis.
- Seek medical care promptly if they suspect an infection, even if symptoms seem mild.

5. Preventing Tick-Borne Diseases

Patients without a spleen are at higher risk of severe complications from infections like babesiosis, a tick-borne illness that can lead to life-threatening complications in asplenic individuals.

- Preventive measures include using insect repellents, wearing protective clothing, and performing regular tick checks after outdoor activities.

6. Medical Alert Identification

Wearing a medical alert bracelet or carrying a card that indicates your asplenic status is highly recommended. This ensures that emergency responders and healthcare providers are aware of your condition and can take appropriate precautions.

7. Lifestyle Adjustments

- Avoiding High-Risk Activities: Contact sports or activities that risk abdominal trauma should be avoided to prevent injury to nearby organs or surgical complications.

- Hygiene Practices: Frequent handwashing and maintaining good hygiene are simple but effective ways to reduce the risk of infections.

The Role of Education and Awareness

A significant part of infection prevention is educating asplenic patients and their families about their increased risk and the importance of proactive measures. Key points include:

- Understanding which symptoms warrant immediate medical attention.

- Keeping track of vaccination schedules and booster doses.

- Recognizing the need for preventive antibiotics and when to use emergency medications.

PART 3: THE SPLENECTOMY PROCEDURE

HOW IS SPLENECTOMY PERFORMED?

Splenectomy, the surgical removal of the spleen, is a procedure performed to treat various medical conditions, ranging from trauma to chronic diseases. The surgery can be done using two main techniques: laparoscopic splenectomy or open splenectomy, depending on the patient's condition and the surgeon's recommendation. Each approach has its benefits and specific considerations, and the choice between them depends on factors like the size of the spleen, the underlying condition, and the urgency of the surgery. Below is a detailed discussion of these techniques, followed by a step-by-step explanation of how the procedure is performed.

*Types of Splenectomy:
Laparoscopic vs. Open Surgery*

1. Laparoscopic Splenectomy

Laparoscopic splenectomy is a minimally invasive surgical technique where the spleen is removed using specialized instruments and a camera inserted through small incisions in the abdomen.

Advantages
- Smaller Incisions: Typically, 3–4 small incisions (less than 1 cm each) are made, resulting in less scarring.

- Reduced Pain: Smaller incisions lead to less post-operative discomfort.
- Faster Recovery: Patients can usually resume normal activities sooner compared to open surgery.
- Lower Risk of Complications: Reduced risk of wound infections and hernias.

Disadvantages
- Limited Field of Vision: Although the laparoscope provides a magnified view, the surgeon's access to certain areas may be restricted.
- Not Suitable for All Cases: Laparoscopic splenectomy may not be feasible for patients with a very large spleen (splenomegaly) or significant scar tissue from previous abdominal surgeries.

2. Open Splenectomy

Open splenectomy is a traditional surgical technique where the spleen is removed through a single large incision in the abdomen.

Advantages
- Better Access: Allows the surgeon to have a direct view and greater control, especially in complex cases such as trauma or cancer.
- Suitable for Larger Spleens: Open surgery is often the preferred method for patients with massively enlarged spleens or severe splenic injuries.
- Preferred in Emergencies: In trauma cases or when there is significant internal bleeding, open surgery is faster and provides better access.

Disadvantages

- Longer Recovery Time: Larger incisions mean a longer healing process and more post-operative discomfort.
- Higher Risk of Complications: There is a greater risk of wound infections and hernias compared to laparoscopic surgery.
- Increased Scarring: The large incision leaves a visible scar.

*Step-by-Step Explanation
of the Procedure*

The surgical procedure for splenectomy involves a series of carefully coordinated steps. While the exact details may vary depending on the surgical approach (laparoscopic or open) and the patient's condition, the general process is as follows:

1. Preoperative Preparation
- Anesthesia: The surgery is performed under general anesthesia. The patient is completely asleep and pain-free during the procedure.
- Positioning: The patient is positioned on their back, with the operating table tilted slightly to the right to improve access to the spleen, which is located in the upper left abdomen.
- Sterilization: The abdominal area is cleaned and sterilized to minimize the risk of infection.

2. Making the Incisions
- Laparoscopic Surgery:

- Small incisions (ports) are made in the abdominal wall.
- A laparoscope (a thin tube with a camera) is inserted through one port, providing a magnified view of the spleen on a monitor.
- Surgical instruments are inserted through the other ports.
- Open Surgery:
- A single large incision (usually 6–12 inches) is made in the upper abdomen, just below the rib cage, to expose the spleen directly.

3. Identifying and Isolating the Spleen

- The surgeon locates the spleen and carefully separates it from surrounding tissues.
- Blood supply to the spleen is managed by isolating and controlling the splenic artery and vein:
- These blood vessels are clamped and divided to prevent bleeding.
- Special surgical clips or sutures are used to seal the vessels.

4. Detaching the Spleen

- The spleen is attached to nearby organs by ligaments (gastrosplenic, splenorenal, and splenocolic ligaments), which are carefully cut or divided to free the spleen.
- During this step, the surgeon must avoid injuring nearby organs, such as the pancreas, stomach, and diaphragm.

5. Removing the Spleen

- Laparoscopic Surgery:
  - The spleen is placed in a specialized retrieval bag and carefully removed through one of the small incisions. For larger spleens, the surgeon may need to break it into smaller pieces within the bag to facilitate removal.
- Open Surgery:
  - The spleen is directly lifted out through the incision.

6. Inspecting the Surgical Area
- The surgeon examines the abdominal cavity for any signs of bleeding or injury to nearby organs.
- In trauma cases, additional steps may be needed to repair damage to surrounding tissues.

7. Closing the Incisions
- Laparoscopic Surgery:
  - The small incisions are closed with dissolvable sutures or surgical glue.
- Open Surgery:
  - The large incision is closed with sutures or staples, and a surgical drain may be placed temporarily to remove excess fluid or blood.

8. Post-Operative Care
- The patient is moved to a recovery area, where they are closely monitored as they wake up from anesthesia.
- Pain management and initial recovery instructions are provided.

Post-Operative Considerations

After the surgery, patients are monitored for complications and supported through their recovery:

Immediate Post-Surgery
- Vital signs (blood pressure, heart rate, oxygen levels) are closely monitored.
- Pain control is managed with medications.
- Patients are encouraged to move and walk as soon as possible to reduce the risk of blood clots and promote healing.

Long-Term Recovery
- Most patients can return to light activities within 2–4 weeks after laparoscopic surgery and 6–8 weeks after open surgery.
- Lifelong preventive measures, such as vaccinations and antibiotics, are critical for infection prevention.

Complications and Risks

While splenectomy is generally safe, it carries some risks, including:
- Bleeding or infection at the surgical site.
- Injury to nearby organs, such as the pancreas or stomach.
- Blood clots (e.g., in the portal vein).
- Long-term risk of overwhelming infections (e.g., sepsis), especially from encapsulated bacteria.

RISKS AND BENEFITS OF SPLENECTOMY

Splenectomy, the surgical removal of the spleen, is a significant procedure with both risks and benefits that must be carefully considered. While the surgery can resolve or manage certain medical conditions effectively, it also has potential short-term and long-term complications, given the spleen's critical role in the immune and circulatory systems.

Surgical Risks and Potential Complications

As with any major surgery, splenectomy carries inherent risks associated with the operation itself, as well as long-term risks arising from the absence of the spleen. These risks can be categorized as immediate (surgical risks) and long-term complications.

1. Surgical Risks
Surgical risks are those that occur during or immediately after the procedure. These risks may vary depending on whether the surgery is performed laparoscopically or as an open procedure.

a. Bleeding
 - The spleen is highly vascular, receiving a significant blood supply from the splenic artery and

vein. During surgery, there is a risk of significant blood loss, particularly if the spleen is enlarged or if there are complications in isolating the blood vessels.

- In some cases, patients may require a blood transfusion during or after surgery.

b. Infection

- Any surgical procedure carries a risk of infection at the incision site or within the abdominal cavity (intra-abdominal infections).
- The use of sterile techniques and prophylactic antibiotics reduces this risk, but patients with a compromised immune system may still be at greater risk.

c. Injury to Nearby Organs

- The spleen is located near several vital organs, including the pancreas, stomach, colon, and diaphragm. Accidental injury to these structures during surgery can lead to complications, such as:
  - Pancreatic leaks or fistulas if the tail of the pancreas is damaged.
  - Perforation of the stomach or bowel, leading to peritonitis.
- These injuries may require additional interventions.

d. Blood Clots

- Post-surgical blood clots, such as deep vein thrombosis (DVT) or portal vein thrombosis, are possible complications. Splenectomy increases the risk of thrombosis due to changes in blood flow and platelet levels.

e. Anesthetic Risks

- General anesthesia carries risks such as allergic reactions, respiratory problems, or cardiovascular events, though these are rare in healthy individuals.

2. Long-Term Complications

The spleen plays a critical role in immunity, and its removal has lifelong implications.

a. Increased Risk of Infections

- Splenectomy increases the risk of severe infections, particularly from encapsulated bacteria such as:
    - Streptococcus pneumoniae (pneumococcus)
    - Haemophilus influenzae type B (Hib)
    - Neisseria meningitidis (meningococcus)
- This condition is known as Overwhelming Post-Splenectomy Infection (OPSI), a rare but life-threatening complication.
- Vaccinations and prophylactic antibiotics are essential to mitigate this risk.

b. Altered Blood Cell Counts

- After splenectomy, platelet levels often increase (thrombocytosis), which can lead to an elevated risk of blood clots in veins or arteries.
- Monitoring platelet levels and, if necessary, using antiplatelet medications can reduce this risk.

c. Long-Term Risk of Thrombosis

- Portal vein thrombosis or splenic vein thrombosis may occur due to changes in blood flow dynamics after splenectomy.
- Chronic conditions like myeloproliferative disorders or cirrhosis further increase this risk.

d. Impaired Immune Function
- The spleen filters blood and removes old or damaged cells, debris, and pathogens. Its absence makes the body less effective at combating certain infections, particularly bloodborne pathogens.
- This immune compromise is especially significant in children, who rely heavily on their spleen for immune function.

Benefits of Splenectomy

While the risks of splenectomy are significant, the procedure can offer substantial benefits for individuals with specific medical conditions. For many patients, splenectomy can improve quality of life, prevent life-threatening complications, and even be curative in some cases.

1. Resolves Underlying Conditions
- Splenectomy can effectively treat conditions where the spleen's function is contributing to disease. For example:
   - In Immune Thrombocytopenic Purpura (ITP): The spleen destroys platelets targeted by the immune system. Removing the spleen halts this process, increasing platelet levels and reducing

bleeding risks.

- In Hereditary Spherocytosis: The spleen disproportionately destroys abnormally shaped red blood cells. Removing it reduces hemolysis, preventing anemia and related complications.

2. Alleviates Symptoms

- In cases of splenomegaly (enlarged spleen), patients often experience pain, discomfort, and early satiety due to pressure on surrounding organs. Splenectomy alleviates these symptoms, improving daily functioning.

- For conditions like portal hypertension, removing the spleen can reduce hypersplenism (overactive spleen), normalizing blood cell counts and improving energy levels.

3. Prevents Life-Threatening Complications

- In traumatic injuries where the spleen is ruptured, immediate splenectomy can prevent fatal internal bleeding.

- In patients with splenic abscesses or cysts, splenectomy removes the source of infection or obstruction, preventing sepsis or other complications.

4. Enhances Efficacy of Cancer Treatment

- In cancers like lymphoma or leukemia that involve the spleen, splenectomy can:
    - Reduce the tumor burden.
    - Improve the effectiveness of chemotherapy or radiation by removing a site of disease involvement.

5. Improves Quality of Life in Chronic Disorders
 - For patients with chronic conditions such as thalassemia major or myelofibrosis, splenectomy can reduce the frequency of transfusions, relieve abdominal discomfort, and improve overall well-being.

Balancing Risks and Benefits

The decision to undergo splenectomy involves weighing the potential risks against the expected benefits. Doctors consider several factors, including:
 - Severity of the Condition: If the spleen's involvement in the disease poses a greater risk than its removal, splenectomy becomes a logical choice.
 - Patient's Age and General Health: Younger patients and those in good health are better able to tolerate surgery and recover from complications.
 - Availability of Alternatives: Non-surgical treatments, such as medications, embolization, or watchful waiting, may be explored before opting for splenectomy.

Mitigating Risks Post-Splenectomy

To maximize the benefits and minimize the risks of splenectomy, patients must adhere to preventive measures, including:
 - Vaccinations: Protect against encapsulated bacteria with pre-surgery and booster doses of

pneumococcal, meningococcal, and Hib vaccines.

- Prophylactic Antibiotics: Daily antibiotics may be prescribed, especially for young children or high-risk patients.

- Prompt Medical Attention: Any signs of infection, such as fever or chills, should be treated as emergencies.

- Lifestyle Adjustments: Avoiding activities that increase infection risk and practicing good hygiene can help prevent complications.

PART 4: LIFE AFTER SPLENECTOMY

YOUR FIRST DAYS AFTER SURGERY

The first few days after splenectomy are critical for your recovery, as your body adjusts to the absence of the spleen and begins to heal from surgery. During this time, you'll be closely monitored by healthcare professionals to ensure that any immediate post-operative challenges are managed effectively. This phase also includes learning how to care for yourself as you transition from the hospital to your home.

What Happens in the Hospital?

After your splenectomy, you will be moved to a recovery area where your vital signs and overall condition are closely monitored. The duration of your hospital stay depends on the type of surgery performed (laparoscopic or open), your overall health, and the presence of any complications.

1. Recovery from Anesthesia
- Waking Up: After surgery, you'll gradually wake up from general anesthesia in a recovery room. Some common experiences include grogginess, nausea, or a sore throat from the breathing tube used during surgery.
- Monitoring: Nurses will monitor your vital signs, including heart rate, blood pressure, oxygen levels, and temperature, to ensure you're stable as you recover from the anesthesia.

- Oxygen Support: If needed, supplemental oxygen may be provided through a nasal cannula or mask until your oxygen levels return to normal.

2. Initial Post-Surgery Assessment
- Pain Management: Pain is expected after surgery, but it will be managed with medications, which may be administered intravenously (IV) or orally. Commonly used pain relievers include acetaminophen, NSAIDs, or opioids for more severe pain.
- Drain and Incision Monitoring: If surgical drains were placed to remove excess fluid or blood, these will be checked regularly to ensure proper functioning. Your surgical incisions will also be inspected for signs of infection or excessive bleeding.

3. Blood Tests and Imaging
- Blood Work: Regular blood tests are performed to monitor your red blood cell count, white blood cell count, platelet levels, and overall recovery.
- Imaging (if needed): In cases of complications or unexpected symptoms, imaging studies like ultrasounds or CT scans may be ordered to assess the surgical site.

4. Movement and Activity
- Getting Out of Bed: Early mobilization is encouraged to prevent complications like blood clots or pneumonia. You may be asked to sit up and even take short walks within a few hours or the day

after surgery, depending on your condition.
- Physical Therapy Support: In some cases, a physical therapist may assist you in regaining mobility safely.

Managing Pain, Drains, and Initial Recovery

1. Managing Pain
Pain management is a crucial aspect of recovery, as it ensures comfort and allows you to move and heal more effectively.

- Types of Pain Relief:
  - IV Pain Medications: Stronger pain medications, such as opioids (e.g., morphine or hydromorphone), are typically given immediately after surgery.
  - Oral Pain Relievers: As your pain decreases, oral medications like acetaminophen or ibuprofen may be used instead.
  - Regional Anesthesia (if used): Some patients receive a nerve block or epidural for pain relief, which provides targeted pain control in the abdominal area.

- Non-Medication Techniques:
  - Deep breathing exercises can help reduce tension and improve oxygenation.
  - Applying a pillow to your abdomen when coughing or moving can minimize pain from the surgical site.

- Expected Pain Levels:

- Pain tends to be more significant after open splenectomy due to the larger incision. Laparoscopic splenectomy generally causes less discomfort, though you may still feel soreness near the incision sites.

2. Managing Surgical Drains

Surgical drains are sometimes placed during splenectomy to remove excess fluid or blood from the surgical site, especially if there was significant bleeding or trauma.

- Function of Drains:
  - These are thin tubes connected to small collection devices that ensure the surgical area remains free of fluid buildup, reducing the risk of infection and promoting healing.

- Care for Drains:
  - Drains are checked regularly by hospital staff to ensure they are functioning properly.
  - The fluid collected in the drains is measured and recorded, providing insight into your healing process.

- Removal of Drains:
  - Drains are typically removed a few days after surgery, once the fluid output decreases significantly. This process is quick and usually causes minimal discomfort.

3. Managing Surgical Incisions

Your surgical incisions will require attention to

prevent infection and ensure proper healing.

- Dressing Changes:
  - Your incisions will be covered with sterile dressings, which are checked and changed regularly by your medical team.

- Signs of Infection:
  - Redness, swelling, warmth, excessive drainage, or fever may indicate an infection. Inform your healthcare provider immediately if you notice these signs.

- Suture or Staple Removal:
  - If non-dissolvable sutures or staples were used, they will typically be removed 7–14 days after surgery.

4. Monitoring for Complications

Although most patients recover without major issues, your medical team will closely watch for potential complications, including:

- Bleeding: Any signs of internal or external bleeding are promptly addressed.
- Infections: Early signs of infection, such as fever or unusual drainage, are treated with antibiotics.
- Blood Clots: You may receive blood-thinning medications or wear compression stockings to reduce the risk of deep vein thrombosis (DVT).
- Pneumonia or Respiratory Issues: Breathing exercises using an incentive spirometer may be encouraged to prevent respiratory complications.

Transitioning to Oral Medications and Eating

Once your condition stabilizes, you'll transition from IV medications to oral pain relievers and other supportive medications. You'll also gradually resume eating and drinking.

- Dietary Progression:
  - Initially, you may be given clear liquids, such as broth or water.
  - As your digestive system resumes normal function, you'll progress to a soft diet and eventually to regular foods.

- Medications:
  - If you require antibiotics or other medications, they will be switched to oral forms before you leave the hospital.

Discharge Planning

Your healthcare team will prepare you for discharge when you meet the following criteria:
- You can eat and drink without nausea.
- Pain is well-controlled with oral medications.
- You can move around safely and perform basic activities, such as walking to the bathroom.
- There are no signs of infection or other complications.

Discharge Instructions

- You'll receive instructions on caring for your incisions, recognizing signs of infection, and managing pain at home.
- You'll also be reminded of follow-up appointments to monitor your recovery.

Emotional and Psychological Recovery

In addition to physical healing, your emotional well-being is important. Many patients feel tired, anxious, or emotional after surgery. Rest and support from family and friends can make this transition easier.

- Coping with Changes:
  - If splenectomy was performed due to trauma or cancer, it may take time to process the experience emotionally.

- Seeking Support:
  - Joining support groups or speaking with a counselor can help you navigate these emotions.

Long-Term Recovery

Recovering from splenectomy is not just about healing from the surgery itself—it also involves adjusting to life without a spleen. This long-term recovery phase requires attention to your physical health, lifestyle adjustments, and a commitment to preventive care to avoid complications such as infections or blood clots. While most individuals recover well and adapt to life without a spleen, understanding the changes and taking the necessary precautions is critical for a healthy future.

ADJUSTING TO LIFE WITHOUT A SPLEEN

The spleen plays a central role in the immune system, filtering blood, removing old or damaged blood cells, and fighting infections caused by certain bacteria. Without a spleen, the body's defenses are compromised, requiring lifelong vigilance to prevent infections and other complications. Adjusting to this new reality involves a combination of medical follow-ups, vaccinations, antibiotics, and lifestyle changes.

1. Increased Risk of Infections
One of the most significant adjustments is managing the increased vulnerability to infections, especially those caused by encapsulated bacteria like Streptococcus pneumoniae, Haemophilus influenzae, and Neisseria meningitidis.

Preventive Measures to Combat Infections
- Vaccinations:
  - Ensuring that you are fully vaccinated is critical. This includes:
    - Pneumococcal vaccines (PCV13 and PPSV23) with periodic booster doses.
    - Meningococcal vaccines (MenACWY and MenB) with regular boosters.
    - Haemophilus influenzae type B (Hib) vaccine.
    - Annual flu vaccine to reduce the risk of

secondary bacterial infections.
- Other vaccines as recommended for travel or regional disease risks (e.g., hepatitis, typhoid, or yellow fever).
- Keep an updated vaccination record, as certain vaccines require boosters every 5–10 years.

- Antibiotic Prophylaxis:
- Some doctors recommend daily prophylactic antibiotics, particularly for children, young adults, or high-risk individuals. This reduces the risk of overwhelming infections, especially in the first few years after surgery.

- Emergency Antibiotics:
- You may be advised to carry a supply of antibiotics for immediate use if you develop symptoms of infection, such as fever or chills, and cannot access medical care promptly.

- Recognizing Infections Early:
- Being vigilant about symptoms such as fever, chills, confusion, or difficulty breathing is essential. These could signal severe infections like sepsis, which requires immediate medical attention.

2. Blood Clot Risk
After splenectomy, platelet levels often rise due to the absence of the spleen's filtering function. This condition, known as thrombocytosis, can increase the risk of blood clots (thrombosis).

Preventive Strategies for Blood Clots

- Regular Monitoring:
  - Your doctor will monitor your platelet levels with regular blood tests in the months following surgery.
- Medications:
  - If platelet levels are very high, antiplatelet medications like aspirin may be prescribed to reduce the risk of clot formation.
- Hydration and Mobility:
  - Staying hydrated and avoiding prolonged periods of immobility, such as sitting for extended periods during travel, can lower the risk of deep vein thrombosis (DVT).

3. Lifestyle Adjustments

Living without a spleen requires certain lifestyle modifications to reduce risks and maintain overall health.

Avoiding High-Risk Activities

- Activities that expose you to injuries or infections should be approached cautiously:
  - Avoid contact sports or activities with a high risk of abdominal trauma, as your body is now more vulnerable to injuries in this area.
  - Wear protective gear (e.g., a seatbelt pad) to protect the abdomen during activities like driving.

Travel Precautions

- Traveling to certain regions, especially those with high risks of malaria, is more complicated for asplenic individuals:
  - Take antimalarial medications if traveling to

endemic areas, as malaria poses a greater risk for people without a spleen.

- Avoid tick-prone areas or take precautions against tick-borne diseases like babesiosis, which can cause severe complications in asplenic individuals.

- Carry an updated medical alert card or wear a bracelet indicating that you are asplenic, so healthcare providers are informed in case of an emergency.

Diet and Exercise
- Maintain a balanced diet rich in vitamins, minerals, and antioxidants to support your immune system.
- Regular exercise helps improve circulation, boosts overall health, and reduces the risk of blood clots.

Gradual Return to Normal Activities

The pace of returning to your daily routine depends on the type of surgery performed (laparoscopic or open splenectomy) and your overall health. While recovery times can vary, most patients can resume normal activities within a few weeks to a few months. The process should be gradual and guided by your body's healing progress.

1. Physical Activity
- First Few Weeks:
  - Avoid strenuous activities or heavy lifting to prevent strain on the surgical site.

- Engage in light activities, such as short walks, to promote circulation and prevent blood clots.
- 4–6 Weeks After Surgery:
  - If you had a laparoscopic splenectomy, you might return to work or school within 2–4 weeks, depending on your energy levels and the nature of your job.
  - For open surgery, this timeline may extend to 6–8 weeks.
- After Full Recovery:
  - Gradually reintroduce exercise routines, starting with low-impact activities like swimming or yoga.
  - Avoid contact sports or high-impact activities unless cleared by your doctor.

2. Work and Daily Responsibilities
- Desk Jobs:
  - Many patients can return to desk jobs within 2–3 weeks after laparoscopic surgery or 4–6 weeks after open surgery.
- Physical Labor:
  - Jobs requiring heavy lifting or physical exertion may require more recovery time. Consult your doctor before resuming such activities.

3. Social Activities
- Socializing and engaging in recreational activities can resume as your energy levels improve, but you should avoid crowded places or environments with a high risk of infections during the initial months.

Follow-Up Care

Regular Check-Ups
- Regular follow-up appointments with your healthcare provider are essential to monitor your recovery and manage any long-term risks.
- Blood tests may be conducted periodically to check for:
  - Platelet levels (to assess the risk of clots).
  - White blood cell counts (to monitor for infections).

Education and Awareness
- Stay informed about your condition and the necessary precautions. Knowing when to seek medical help and staying up-to-date on vaccinations are crucial aspects of long-term care.

Psychological Adjustment

Adapting to life without a spleen can be emotionally challenging for some patients, especially those who underwent the surgery unexpectedly due to trauma or a sudden medical condition.

- Dealing with Anxiety:
  - It's natural to feel anxious about your increased vulnerability to infections or the need for lifelong precautions. Speaking with a counselor or joining a support group can help.
- Support Networks:
  - Family and friends can play a significant role in emotional recovery. Share your concerns with loved ones and involve them in your care plan.

PREVENTING AND MANAGING INFECTIONS

The spleen plays a critical role in the immune system by filtering blood, removing pathogens, and facilitating the production of antibodies to fight infections. After splenectomy, the absence of the spleen (asplenia) compromises the body's ability to defend against certain types of infections, especially those caused by encapsulated bacteria. As a result, individuals without a spleen are at an increased risk of severe infections, including life-threatening conditions like sepsis.

Risks of Infections Due to Asplenia

1. Increased Susceptibility to Encapsulated Bacteria
Encapsulated bacteria are particularly dangerous for asplenic individuals because the spleen plays a key role in producing antibodies and activating immune cells to fight these pathogens. The primary bacteria of concern include:
- Streptococcus pneumoniae (pneumococcus): Can cause pneumonia, meningitis, or bloodstream infections (sepsis).
- Haemophilus influenzae type B (Hib): Causes respiratory infections, meningitis, and sepsis.
- Neisseria meningitidis (meningococcus): Causes meningitis and bloodstream infections.

2. Overwhelming Post-Splenectomy Infection (OPSI)

- OPSI is a rare but life-threatening condition characterized by rapid onset and progression of sepsis. It occurs due to the body's inability to control bacterial infections effectively without the spleen.
- OPSI has a high mortality rate if not treated promptly, making early recognition and prevention critical.

3. Risk of Other Infections

Asplenic individuals are also more susceptible to other infections, including:

- Tick-Borne Diseases: Infections like babesiosis can be severe in asplenic patients.
- Malaria: Without a spleen, the body struggles to filter malaria parasites, leading to higher disease severity.
- Viral Infections: Some viral infections, such as influenza, can predispose asplenic patients to secondary bacterial infections.

4. Risk Factors Increasing Infection Susceptibility

- Age: Children and older adults are more vulnerable to infections post-splenectomy.
- Underlying Conditions: Comorbidities such as diabetes, cancer, or autoimmune diseases further increase infection risks.

Preventive Strategies to Reduce Infection Risks

Preventive care is the cornerstone of infection

management in asplenic individuals. These strategies significantly reduce the risk of infections and improve long-term outcomes.

1. Vaccinations

Vaccinations are essential for asplenic patients and should be administered according to recommended guidelines.

- Key Vaccines:
  - Pneumococcal Vaccines:
    - PCV13 (Prevnar 13): Provides protection against 13 pneumococcal strains.
    - PPSV23 (Pneumovax 23): Protects against an additional 23 pneumococcal strains. Boosters are required every 5 years.
  - Meningococcal Vaccines:
    - MenACWY: Protects against meningococcal groups A, C, W, and Y. Boosters are given every 5 years.
    - MenB: Protects against meningococcal group B and requires a two-dose schedule.
  - Haemophilus Influenzae Type B (Hib):
    - A single dose is recommended if not already vaccinated.
  - Influenza Vaccine:
    - Annual flu shots are essential to prevent viral infections that can lead to secondary bacterial complications.
  - COVID-19 Vaccine:
    - Full vaccination and booster doses are advised to reduce the risk of severe illness.

- Travel Vaccines:
  - Vaccinations for typhoid, hepatitis A and B, yellow fever, and others may be recommended for travel to certain regions.

- Timing of Vaccinations:
  - Ideally, vaccines should be given 2–4 weeks before elective splenectomy. If surgery is urgent, vaccinations should be administered as soon as the patient has recovered.

2. Prophylactic Antibiotics
- Daily antibiotics are often recommended, particularly for high-risk individuals, such as young children or those with a history of severe infections.
- Common Antibiotics:
  - Penicillin V or amoxicillin for daily use.
  - Alternatives such as azithromycin or erythromycin for those allergic to penicillin.
- Antibiotics are typically used for at least the first 2 years after surgery, but some individuals may require lifelong prophylaxis.

3. Emergency Antibiotics
- Asplenic individuals are often advised to carry a supply of antibiotics to take immediately if symptoms of infection develop, particularly when medical care is not immediately accessible.

4. Hygiene and Lifestyle Measures
- Handwashing: Regular handwashing with soap is one of the simplest and most effective ways to prevent infections.

- Oral Hygiene: Good dental care reduces the risk of infections that could spread from the mouth to the bloodstream.
- Food Safety: Avoid raw or undercooked meats, unpasteurized dairy products, and other high-risk foods.
- Avoiding Animal Bites: Seek prompt treatment for animal bites or scratches, which can introduce harmful bacteria like Capnocytophaga canimorsus.

5. Avoiding High-Risk Activities
- Travel Precautions: Prevent exposure to diseases like malaria by using insect repellents, wearing protective clothing, and taking antimalarial medications if traveling to endemic areas.
- Protective Clothing: Wear gloves when gardening or working outdoors to avoid cuts and scratches.

6. Medical Alert Identification
- Wearing a medical alert bracelet or carrying a card indicating asplenia is essential. This helps healthcare providers take immediate, appropriate measures in case of illness or injury.

Recognizing Signs of Severe Infections

Despite the best preventive measures, infections can still occur in asplenic individuals. Early recognition of symptoms is critical for timely treatment and preventing complications.

1. Common Signs of Infection
- Fever (temperature above 100.4°F or 38°C)

- Chills or shivering
- Rapid heart rate or breathing
- Fatigue or weakness
- Nausea or vomiting
- Skin rash or redness around a wound

2. Signs of Severe Infections or Sepsis

Sepsis is a life-threatening complication that occurs when an infection spreads throughout the body, triggering an extreme immune response. Warning signs include:
- Confusion or altered mental state
- Severe difficulty breathing
- Low blood pressure or dizziness
- Extreme weakness or inability to stay awake
- Cold, clammy, or pale skin
- Bluish discoloration of lips or fingertips

3. When to Seek Medical Help
- Seek immediate medical attention if:
  - You have a fever above 100.4°F that does not resolve quickly.
  - You experience any of the severe symptoms listed above.
  - You feel unwell and suspect an infection, even if symptoms seem mild initially.

4. Emergency Protocols
- Inform the medical team about your asplenia status to ensure appropriate treatment.
- Antibiotics are often started immediately, even before test results confirm the infection, to reduce

the risk of sepsis.

Post-Infection Follow-Up

- If you have been treated for an infection, follow up with your healthcare provider to ensure full recovery and adjust preventive measures as needed.
- Regular health check-ups and vaccinations remain crucial to prevent future infections.

FOLLOW-UP CARE

Follow-up care is a critical component of recovery and long-term health after splenectomy. While the immediate post-operative period focuses on physical healing, follow-up care extends far beyond wound recovery. It involves monitoring for complications, managing lifelong health risks, and implementing strategies to prevent infections and other potential issues associated with living without a spleen. Effective follow-up care ensures that patients can live healthy and fulfilling lives, even with the challenges posed by asplenia.

Key Components of Follow-Up Care

1. Regular Medical Check-Ups
Routine follow-up visits with your healthcare provider are essential to monitor your recovery and manage potential complications. These visits typically include:
- Physical Examination:
  - Assessment of the surgical site for proper healing.
  - Checking for signs of infection, swelling, or other abnormalities.
- Blood Tests:
  - Monitoring platelet levels to identify thrombocytosis (elevated platelet count), which can increase the risk of blood clots.
  - Checking white blood cell counts to assess

immune system function.
- Vital Signs Monitoring:
  - Regular monitoring of blood pressure, heart rate, and temperature to detect any signs of underlying issues.

2. Long-Term Monitoring for Complications

Splenectomy is associated with specific long-term risks that require ongoing vigilance:

- Thrombocytosis:
  - The spleen normally helps regulate platelet levels. After splenectomy, platelet levels may rise significantly, increasing the risk of blood clots (thrombosis) in veins or arteries.
  - Regular blood tests are necessary to monitor platelet counts. If levels are too high, your doctor may prescribe antiplatelet medications such as aspirin to reduce clotting risks.
- Infections:
  - Asplenic individuals are at higher risk of severe infections, particularly from encapsulated bacteria. Regular follow-ups ensure that vaccinations are up to date and that any signs of infection are addressed promptly.

3. Vaccination Maintenance

Vaccinations are a cornerstone of follow-up care for asplenic patients. While many vaccines are administered before or shortly after surgery, booster doses and additional vaccines are required to maintain immunity.

- Pneumococcal Vaccines:
  - Booster doses of PPSV23 (Pneumovax 23) are recommended every 5 years to protect against pneumococcal infections.
- Meningococcal Vaccines:
  - Regular boosters for MenACWY (every 5 years) and MenB (as per schedule) are necessary.
- Annual Influenza Vaccine:
  - The flu shot is critical for preventing influenza, which can predispose individuals to secondary bacterial infections.
- COVID-19 Vaccines:
  - Keep up with the latest recommendations for booster doses to ensure protection against COVID-19.
- Travel Vaccines:
  - Depending on travel destinations, additional vaccines (e.g., yellow fever, typhoid, hepatitis A and B) may be required.

Preventive Strategies and Lifestyle Modifications

1. Prophylactic Antibiotics

Prophylactic antibiotics are often prescribed to reduce the risk of infections, particularly in the first few years after surgery or for individuals with a history of severe infections.

- Daily Antibiotics:
  - Penicillin or amoxicillin is commonly prescribed

for daily use. Alternatives like erythromycin may be used for those allergic to penicillin.
- Emergency Antibiotics:
  - Asplenic individuals are advised to carry a supply of antibiotics to start immediately if they develop symptoms of infection, particularly in situations where medical care may not be readily available.

2. Recognizing Early Signs of Infection

Part of effective follow-up care involves educating patients to recognize the early signs of infection and respond promptly. These include:
- Fever above 100.4°F (38°C).
- Chills, shivering, or sweating.
- Fatigue or weakness.
- Confusion or altered mental state.
- Rapid breathing or heart rate.
- Skin rash or redness around a wound.

Patients are advised to seek medical attention immediately if these symptoms occur, as infections in asplenic individuals can escalate rapidly into sepsis.

3. Lifestyle Adjustments

Follow-up care also includes guidance on lifestyle changes to minimize health risks:
- Avoiding High-Risk Activities:
  - Activities that carry a high risk of cuts, scrapes, or bites (e.g., gardening, animal handling) should be approached with caution.
  - Contact sports or other activities that could cause

abdominal trauma are discouraged.
- Travel Precautions:
  - Travelers should take precautions against diseases like malaria and tick-borne illnesses, as asplenic individuals are more susceptible to severe complications.
  - Antimalarial medications, insect repellents, and protective clothing are essential for travel to endemic regions.
- Healthy Diet and Exercise:
  - A balanced diet and regular exercise promote overall health and help prevent conditions like obesity and cardiovascular disease.

Monitoring Mental and Emotional Well-Being

Living without a spleen can bring psychological challenges, including anxiety about infection risks or adjusting to a new lifestyle. Follow-up care should address mental health needs as well:
- Counseling or Therapy:
  - Professional support can help patients cope with anxiety or stress related to their condition.
- Support Groups:
  - Connecting with others who have undergone splenectomy can provide valuable emotional support and practical advice.
- Education:
  - Providing patients and their families with accurate information about asplenia and its

management can alleviate fears and empower them to take control of their health.

Emergency Preparedness

As part of follow-up care, asplenic individuals are encouraged to prepare for emergencies:
- Medical Alert Identification:
  - Wearing a medical alert bracelet or carrying a card that indicates asplenia helps healthcare providers respond appropriately in emergencies.
- Emergency Antibiotic Supply:
  - Having a readily available supply of antibiotics ensures that treatment can begin immediately if symptoms of infection develop.

Special Considerations for Children

Children who have undergone splenectomy require extra attention during follow-up care:
- Vaccination Compliance:
  - Children need to follow an age-appropriate vaccination schedule, including boosters, to maintain immunity.
- Growth and Development Monitoring:
  - Regular check-ups ensure that they are meeting developmental milestones and that no complications from splenectomy are interfering with their overall health.

Follow-Up Frequency and Duration

The frequency of follow-up visits may vary

depending on the individual's age, underlying health condition, and time elapsed since surgery:
- First Year After Surgery:
  - Follow-up appointments are more frequent (every 1–3 months) to monitor recovery and ensure that vaccinations and antibiotics are effective.
- Long-Term Follow-Up:
  - After the first year, visits may be scheduled annually, with additional check-ups as needed for vaccination boosters, new symptoms, or travel planning.

Long-Term Outlook

With proper follow-up care, most individuals adapt well to life without a spleen and maintain good health. The key to a positive long-term outlook lies in proactive management of infection risks, adherence to vaccination schedules, and maintaining a healthy lifestyle. Regular communication with healthcare providers ensures that any new risks or challenges are addressed promptly.

PART 5: LIVING WELL WITHOUT A SPLEEN

DIET, EXERCISE, AND LIFESTYLE TIPS

Adjusting to life without a spleen involves adopting a healthy lifestyle to support your immune system and overall well-being. After splenectomy, the body becomes more vulnerable to certain infections, and the immune system requires additional care to function optimally. A well-balanced diet, regular physical activity, and mindful lifestyle choices can significantly improve your quality of life and reduce health risks. By focusing on nourishing foods, staying active, and making protective changes to your daily routine, you can maintain long-term health and vitality.

Nutrition is one of the most important aspects of immune health. Eating a balanced diet that includes a variety of nutrient-dense foods supports your body's defenses and overall recovery. Fruits and vegetables, especially those rich in vitamins A, C, and E, play a vital role in maintaining immune function. Brightly colored produce such as spinach, kale, bell peppers, oranges, and berries contains powerful antioxidants that help combat oxidative stress and strengthen the immune response. Protein is another cornerstone of immune support, as it aids in cell repair and the production of antibodies. Lean meats, fish, eggs, and legumes are excellent sources of protein, while fatty fish like salmon provide omega-3 fatty acids, which reduce inflammation. Whole grains like quinoa, brown rice, and oats provide essential nutrients and sustained energy, helping the body recover and maintain its strength. Additionally, nuts and seeds, particularly almonds, walnuts, and sunflower seeds, are rich in healthy fats, zinc, and selenium, all of which contribute to a healthy immune system.

Hydration is equally crucial for overall health and immune function. Drinking plenty of water throughout the day helps the body flush out toxins and supports the circulation of immune cells. Incorporating probiotics through foods like yogurt, kefir, or fermented vegetables such as kimchi and sauerkraut can improve gut health, which plays a significant role in immune activity. Limiting processed foods, sugary snacks, and beverages is advisable, as they can weaken the immune system and contribute to inflammation. Practicing good food hygiene is also essential for asplenic individuals to avoid foodborne illnesses. Washing fruits and vegetables thoroughly, cooking meats to safe temperatures, and avoiding unpasteurized dairy products or undercooked seafood can minimize exposure to harmful bacteria.

Exercise is another key component of maintaining health after splenectomy. Regular physical activity improves circulation, which helps immune cells move efficiently throughout the body to detect and combat infections. Low-impact exercises, such as walking, swimming, or yoga, are particularly beneficial during the recovery phase and beyond. These activities strengthen the cardiovascular system, enhance flexibility, and improve mental well-being without putting excessive strain on the body. As strength and stamina improve, incorporating light strength training or resistance exercises can help build muscle and bone density. Activities like cycling or dancing can be gradually reintroduced to boost endurance and maintain a healthy weight. However, asplenic individuals should avoid high-impact or contact sports that carry a risk of abdominal trauma. If engaging in such activities is unavoidable, wearing protective gear can reduce the risk of injury.

Returning to exercise after surgery requires patience and a gradual approach. In the first few weeks post-surgery, focus on gentle movements like short walks or light stretching to encourage circulation and reduce the risk of blood clots. Over time, you can increase the duration and intensity of your workouts as your body heals. Listening to your body is essential; if you experience pain, fatigue, or discomfort during or after exercise, consult your doctor before continuing. Consistency is important, and even small amounts of physical activity can significantly improve overall health and immune resilience.

Lifestyle adjustments are equally important in maintaining long-term health. Sleep is a foundational aspect of recovery and immune function. Aim for seven to nine hours of quality sleep each night to allow your body to repair and regenerate. Establishing a consistent sleep schedule, avoiding screens before bedtime, and creating a calming nighttime routine can improve sleep quality. Managing stress is another critical factor. Chronic stress can weaken the immune system, making the body more susceptible to infections. Practices such as meditation, deep breathing, journaling, or engaging in enjoyable hobbies can help reduce stress levels. Regular exercise also contributes to emotional well-being by releasing endorphins and reducing anxiety.

Preventive measures play a vital role in protecting asplenic individuals from infections. Maintaining good hygiene, such as frequent handwashing and proper oral care, can prevent the spread of harmful bacteria. Avoiding smoking and limiting alcohol consumption further support immune health and reduce the risk of chronic illnesses. Travel requires special precautions, particularly when visiting regions where diseases like malaria or typhoid are prevalent. Using insect repellents, wearing protective clothing, and taking prescribed antimalarial medications can reduce risks. Before traveling, consult a healthcare provider to ensure you are adequately vaccinated and prepared for the trip.

Incorporating these dietary, exercise, and lifestyle

practices into your daily routine can make a profound difference in your overall health and well-being. While living without a spleen presents unique challenges, adopting a proactive approach to your health empowers you to reduce risks and lead a vibrant, fulfilling life.

TRAVELING AND SPECIAL CONSIDERATIONS

Traveling after splenectomy requires thoughtful planning and precautions to ensure your health and safety, especially when visiting regions with heightened risks of infection or specific diseases. The absence of a spleen increases your susceptibility to severe infections, so taking preventive measures is essential. With proper preparation and awareness, you can enjoy your travels while minimizing potential risks.

One of the most critical considerations for international travel is protecting yourself against region-specific infections, particularly those transmitted by insects. For example, malaria poses a significant threat to asplenic individuals because the spleen plays a crucial role in filtering and combating the parasites responsible for the disease. Without this defense mechanism, malaria infections can progress rapidly and become life-threatening. If you plan to visit a malaria-endemic area, consult your healthcare provider well in advance. Antimalarial medications such as atovaquone-proguanil, doxycycline, or mefloquine can significantly reduce your risk. It is essential to start taking these medications before entering the region and continue as directed, even after leaving, to ensure complete protection. In addition to medication, use physical barriers to avoid mosquito bites, such as sleeping under insecticide-treated bed nets, wearing long-sleeved clothing and long pants, and applying a reliable insect repellent containing DEET or picaridin to exposed skin.

Carrying a supply of emergency antibiotics is another crucial aspect of travel preparation. Asplenic individuals are at higher risk of overwhelming infections, which can develop rapidly and require immediate treatment. Discuss with your doctor the specific antibiotics to include in your travel kit, such as amoxicillin-clavulanate or azithromycin, which can be taken at the first sign of an infection if medical care is not immediately accessible. These medications act as a safeguard, especially in remote areas where prompt access to healthcare facilities may be limited. Be sure to familiarize yourself with the symptoms of infections, such as fever, chills, and fatigue, and start antibiotics promptly while seeking medical assistance.

Updating your vaccinations is equally critical before traveling, particularly when visiting areas with vaccine-preventable diseases. Asplenic individuals should ensure that their regular vaccinations, such as pneumococcal, meningococcal, and Haemophilus influenzae type B (Hib), are current, as these provide protection against encapsulated bacteria. In addition to routine vaccines, travel-specific vaccinations may be required depending on your destination. For instance, if you are traveling to areas where yellow fever is endemic, you may need a yellow fever vaccine, although some countries require documentation of this vaccination for entry. Other important travel vaccines include typhoid, hepatitis A and B, Japanese encephalitis, and rabies. Plan your travel well in advance to allow enough time to complete any multi-dose vaccine schedules or to recover from possible vaccine side effects.

Carrying a medical alert bracelet or identification card indicating your asplenic status is an important safety measure during travel. In the event of a medical emergency, healthcare providers need to know about your condition to provide appropriate and timely treatment. The identification should clearly state that you are asplenic and outline critical information, such as your heightened risk of infections and any allergies or medications you are taking. This small step can make a significant difference in ensuring that you receive effective care, especially in unfamiliar healthcare systems.

Beyond vaccinations and medications, practical hygiene measures are vital to staying healthy while traveling. Hand hygiene is one of the simplest yet most effective ways to prevent infections. Carry an alcohol-based hand sanitizer for situations where soap and water are unavailable. Pay close attention to food and water safety, as contaminated food or drinks can introduce harmful bacteria and parasites. Avoid raw or undercooked foods, unpasteurized dairy products, and untreated water or ice. Instead, choose bottled or boiled water and freshly cooked meals served hot. These precautions are especially important in regions with poor sanitation or where foodborne illnesses are common.

When traveling to areas with high exposure to animals, such as rural or wilderness destinations, take extra precautions to avoid bites and scratches. Animal bites can introduce harmful bacteria like Capnocytophaga canimorsus, which can cause severe infections in asplenic individuals. Avoid handling stray or wild animals, and seek medical attention promptly if you are bitten or scratched. In some cases, you may need prophylactic antibiotics or even post-exposure vaccinations, such as for rabies.

Travel insurance is another key consideration for asplenic travelers. Ensure that your insurance policy includes coverage for medical emergencies, including hospitalization and evacuation, in case you require advanced treatment while abroad. Having access to a reliable healthcare provider network can alleviate stress and provide peace of mind during your trip.

Proper preparation also includes packing essential medical supplies. In addition to antibiotics and medications, bring any prescribed prophylactic antibiotics, a thermometer for monitoring fever, and a first-aid kit with items such as bandages, antiseptic wipes, and pain relievers. These supplies ensure you are equipped to handle minor health issues without delay. Keep your medications in their original labeled packaging and carry a copy of your prescriptions to avoid issues with customs or border control.

While traveling, remain vigilant about your health. Monitor for signs of infection, such as fever, chills, shortness of breath, or unexplained fatigue, and seek medical care immediately if symptoms arise. Many asplenic individuals find it helpful to research local healthcare facilities at their destination before departure to ensure they know where to go in an emergency. Staying informed and prepared empowers you to respond effectively to potential health challenges, minimizing risks and ensuring a safe and enjoyable trip.

CHILDREN AND SPLENECTOMY

Splenectomy in children presents unique challenges and requires a tailored approach to their care and monitoring. While the procedure is sometimes necessary to manage specific conditions, such as hereditary spherocytosis, immune thrombocytopenic purpura (ITP), or trauma, its impact on a child's developing immune system demands careful attention. Ensuring adequate care and regular follow-up as they grow is essential to minimize risks and support their overall health and development.

The spleen plays a vital role in a child's immune system, particularly during the early years when their immune defenses are still maturing. Without a spleen, children are at an increased risk of life-threatening infections caused by encapsulated bacteria, such as Streptococcus pneumoniae, Haemophilus influenzae type B (Hib), and Neisseria meningitidis. This heightened vulnerability requires rigorous preventive measures, beginning with an age-appropriate vaccination schedule. Vaccines serve as the cornerstone of protection, and pediatric patients undergoing splenectomy must receive pneumococcal, meningococcal, and Hib vaccines well before surgery if possible. These vaccines provide immunity against the most common pathogens that pose a threat to asplenic individuals, and booster doses are critical to maintaining protection as the child grows. For children unable to receive pre-surgery vaccinations due to the urgency of the procedure, post-operative immunization should be initiated as soon as they recover sufficiently.

In addition to vaccinations, children who have undergone splenectomy often benefit from prophylactic antibiotics to prevent severe infections during the years when their immune systems are most at risk. Daily doses of penicillin or amoxicillin are commonly prescribed for younger children, particularly those under the age of five, as their ability to fight infections remains underdeveloped. These antibiotics serve as a safety net, reducing the likelihood of bacterial infections that could progress rapidly. Depending on the child's overall health and the specific circumstances of their splenectomy, some pediatric patients may require lifelong antibiotic prophylaxis. For children allergic to penicillin, alternatives such as erythromycin are typically used. Parents and caregivers must also be educated on the importance of adherence to these preventive treatments to ensure their child's safety.

Monitoring a child's health post-splenectomy involves more than just infection prevention. Regular medical check-ups are essential to track their growth and development while addressing any complications that may arise. Blood tests are often conducted to monitor platelet levels, as thrombocytosis (elevated platelet counts) is a common occurrence after splenectomy. High platelet levels increase the risk of blood clots, which can lead to severe complications if left unchecked. In some cases, antiplatelet medications such as low-dose aspirin may be recommended to mitigate this risk. Physicians also monitor the child's overall immune function, ensuring that their vaccination record remains up to date and that booster doses are administered as needed to maintain immunity.

Children without a spleen require ongoing education about their condition as they grow older, transitioning from parental management to self-care. This gradual process ensures that they understand the importance of preventive measures, such as recognizing early signs of infection and seeking prompt medical attention. Teaching children to take responsibility for their health helps them navigate the challenges of asplenia with confidence and independence. For example, they should learn to carry a supply of emergency antibiotics, which can be taken at the first sign of illness while seeking medical care. Additionally, wearing a medical alert bracelet or carrying an identification card that indicates their asplenic status is essential, as it informs healthcare providers of their condition in emergencies and ensures timely, appropriate treatment.

Hygiene and lifestyle practices also play a significant

role in protecting asplenic children. Parents should encourage good habits, such as regular handwashing with soap and water, to minimize exposure to harmful bacteria. Proper oral hygiene is equally important, as infections originating in the mouth can spread to other parts of the body. When it comes to dietary habits, children should avoid raw or undercooked foods, particularly meats and eggs, to reduce the risk of foodborne illnesses. Families should also be vigilant about animal bites or scratches, which can introduce dangerous bacteria like Capnocytophaga canimorsus. Any animal-related injuries should be cleaned thoroughly, and medical attention should be sought promptly.

As asplenic children grow, certain activities and travel plans may require additional precautions. Parents should consult healthcare providers before international travel, as some destinations may pose heightened risks of exposure to diseases like malaria or typhoid. Prophylactic antimalarial medications, insect repellents, and protective clothing are essential for travel to malaria-endemic areas. Additional vaccinations, such as those for yellow fever or Japanese encephalitis, may also be recommended based on the travel itinerary. When participating in sports or physical activities, children should avoid contact sports that could result in abdominal trauma. If they wish to engage in such activities, protective gear can help minimize risks.

Emotional and psychological support is another critical aspect of care for children who have undergone splenectomy. The need for lifelong precautions and the awareness of their heightened infection risk can be overwhelming, particularly for older children and teenagers. Parents and caregivers should foster open communication, allowing the child to express their concerns and fears. Support groups for families of asplenic children can provide valuable resources, shared experiences, and emotional reassurance. For children experiencing significant anxiety or emotional challenges, professional counseling can help them develop coping strategies and build resilience.

A LETTER TO THE READER

Dear Reader,

Life without a spleen may seem daunting, but it is neither a sentence of frailty nor a barrier to living with strength and purpose. You may feel as though something vital has been taken from you—a cornerstone of your physical health dismantled. But let me remind you: you are not defined by the loss of an organ. Instead, you are defined by your capacity to adapt, to confront challenges with courage, and to embrace the discipline and responsibility required to thrive.

The world is not a safe place, and your condition underscores that reality in ways most people never have to contemplate. But herein lies an opportunity. You can face this new reality with your eyes wide open, prepared to act with vigilance and resolve. Knowledge is your greatest ally now. You understand the risks that come with asplenia—greater susceptibility to infections, the need for vaccinations, the importance of lifestyle adjustments—and this understanding arms you against complacency. To live well without a spleen is to live deliberately, aware of the steps you must take to protect yourself and, more importantly, why you must take them.

Take responsibility for your health. Keep your vaccinations up to date—not because someone else tells you to, but because you recognize that this is a practical and meaningful way to protect yourself and those who depend on you. Maintain a balanced diet and stay active, not simply for the sake of appearance or arbitrary notions of fitness, but because a strong body and resilient mind are the foundation of a fulfilling life. Carry emergency antibiotics and wear a medical alert bracelet—not out of fear, but as a reflection of your commitment to preparedness and self-care. In doing these things, you create order in the chaos of an unpredictable world.

But let us not stop at survival. Thriving after splenectomy is not merely about avoiding danger; it is about finding the courage to fully participate in life despite its risks. Travel, explore, connect with others, and pursue your goals with determination. Do not let the absence of an organ diminish the presence of your ambition. You are not fragile. You are adaptable. You have already overcome the surgery, the recovery, and the initial shock of adjustment. What lies ahead is not limitation but opportunity—the chance to redefine what health and strength mean to you.

Remember that you are not alone. There are others who share your challenges, and they, too, are striving to live well. Seek them out, share your experiences, and learn from theirs. Human beings are social creatures, and it is in community and connection that we find our greatest resilience.

Finally, do not dwell in bitterness over what has been lost. Instead, focus on what you can build in its place. The loss of your spleen is not the loss of your agency, your will, or your capacity to grow. It is a call to action—a demand to be more vigilant, more intentional, and more engaged in the process of living. In answering that call, you will discover not only how to thrive after splenectomy but also how to thrive as a human being in a world that is always uncertain.

You have the tools. You have the knowledge. Now, take up the responsibility, and live your life with purpose.

Sincerely,
Dr. Bhratri Bhushan, MD, DM

ABOUT THE AUTHOR

Dr. Bhratri Bhushan

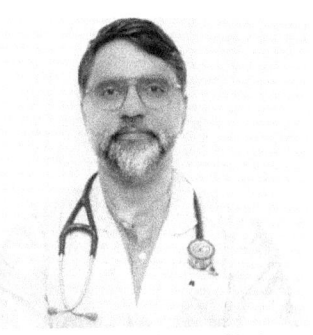

Dr. Bhratri Bhushan is a consultant medical oncologist and hematologist. He has a rich academic and research background, having published more than two hundred books on the subjects of oncology and internal medicine. His scholarly contributions have been featured in renowned journals of medical literature. For a comprehensive collection of his works, please visit his AuthorCentral page at www.amazon.com/author/bhratribhushan

www.ingramcontent.com/pod-product-compliance
Lightning Source LLC
Chambersburg PA
CBHW070152230526
45471CB00002B/624